THIS LOG BOOK ORGANIZER BELONGS TO

_____

{PERSONAL INFORMATION & INSURANCE LOG SHEET}

NAME:	
ADDRESS:	
DATE OF BIRTH	
PHONE NUMBER	
SOCIAL SECURITY	

{PRIMARY HEALTH INSURANCE}	
INSURED'S NAME:	
INSURANCE COMPANY NAME	
MEMBER 1.D. #	
POLICY NUMBER	
GROUP NUMBER	

{SECONDARY HEALTH INSURANCE}	
INSURED'S NAME:	
INSURANCE COMPANY NAME	
MEMBER 1.D. #	
POLICY NUMBER	
GROUP NUMBER	

{PERSONAL INFORMATION & INSURANCE LOG SHEET}

NAME:	
ADDRESS:	
DATE OF BIRTH	
PHONE NUMBER	
SOCIAL SECURITY	

{PRIMARY HEALTH INSURANCE}	
INSURED'S NAME:	
INSURANCE COMPANY NAME	
MEMBER 1.D. #	
POLICY NUMBER	
GROUP NUMBER	

{SECONDARY HEALTH INSURANCE}	
INSURED'S NAME:	
INSURANCE COMPANY NAME	
MEMBER 1.D. #	
POLICY NUMBER	
GROUP NUMBER	

{PERSONAL INFORMATION & INSURANCE LOG SHEET}

NAME:	
ADDRESS:	
DATE OF BIRTH	
PHONE NUMBER	
SOCIAL SECURITY	

{PRIMARY HEALTH INSURANCE}	
INSURED'S NAME:	
INSURANCE COMPANY NAME	
MEMBER 1.D. #	
POLICY NUMBER	
GROUP NUMBER	

{SECONDARY HEALTH INSURANCE}	
INSURED'S NAME:	
INSURANCE COMPANY NAME	
MEMBER 1.D. #	
POLICY NUMBER	
GROUP NUMBER	

{PERSONAL INFORMATION & INSURANCE LOG SHEET}

NAME:	
ADDRESS:	
DATE OF BIRTH	
PHONE NUMBER	
SOCIAL SECURITY	

{PRIMARY HEALTH INSURANCE}	
INSURED'S NAME:	
INSURANCE COMPANY NAME	
MEMBER 1.D. #	
POLICY NUMBER	
GROUP NUMBER	

{SECONDARY HEALTH INSURANCE}	
INSURED'S NAME:	
INSURANCE COMPANY NAME	
MEMBER 1.D. #	
POLICY NUMBER	
GROUP NUMBER	

{PERSONAL INFORMATION & INSURANCE LOG SHEET}

NAME:	
ADDRESS:	
DATE OF BIRTH	
PHONE NUMBER	
SOCIAL SECURITY	

{PRIMARY HEALTH INSURANCE}	
INSURED'S NAME:	
INSURANCE COMPANY NAME	
MEMBER 1.D. #	
POLICY NUMBER	
GROUP NUMBER	

{SECONDARY HEALTH INSURANCE}	
INSURED'S NAME:	
INSURANCE COMPANY NAME	
MEMBER 1.D. #	
POLICY NUMBER	
GROUP NUMBER	

{PERSONAL EMERGENCY CONTACT LIST}

NAME:	
ADDRESS:	
PHONE:	
RELATIONSHIP:	

NAME:	
ADDRESS:	
PHONE:	
RELATIONSHIP:	

NAME:	
ADDRESS:	
PHONE:	
RELATIONSHIP:	

NAME:	
ADDRESS:	
PHONE:	
RELATIONSHIP:	

{PERSONAL EMERGENCY CONTACT LIST}

NAME:	
ADDRESS:	
PHONE:	
RELATIONSHIP:	

NAME:	
ADDRESS:	
PHONE:	
RELATIONSHIP:	

NAME:	
ADDRESS:	
PHONE:	
RELATIONSHIP:	

NAME:	
ADDRESS:	
PHONE:	
RELATIONSHIP:	

{PERSONAL EMERGENCY CONTACT LIST}

NAME:	
ADDRESS:	
PHONE:	
RELATIONSHIP:	

NAME:	
ADDRESS:	
PHONE:	
RELATIONSHIP:	

NAME:	
ADDRESS:	
PHONE:	
RELATIONSHIP:	

NAME:	
ADDRESS:	
PHONE:	
RELATIONSHIP:	

{PERSONAL EMERGENCY CONTACT LIST}

NAME:	
ADDRESS:	
PHONE:	
RELATIONSHIP:	

NAME:	
ADDRESS:	
PHONE:	
RELATIONSHIP:	

NAME:	
ADDRESS:	
PHONE:	
RELATIONSHIP:	

NAME:	
ADDRESS:	
PHONE:	
RELATIONSHIP:	

{PERSONAL EMERGENCY CONTACT LIST}

NAME:	
ADDRESS:	
PHONE:	
RELATIONSHIP:	

NAME:	
ADDRESS:	
PHONE:	
RELATIONSHIP:	

NAME:	
ADDRESS:	
PHONE:	
RELATIONSHIP:	

NAME:	
ADDRESS:	
PHONE:	
RELATIONSHIP:	

{PHYSICIAN CONTACT LIST}

Specialty:
Name:
Address:
Phone Number:
Fax Number:

Specialty:
Name:
Address:
Phone Number:
Fax Number:

Specialty:
Name:
Address:
Phone Number:
Fax Number:

Specialty:
Name:
Address:
Phone Number:
Fax Number:

{PHYSICIAN CONTACT LIST}

Specialty:
Name:
Address:
Phone Number:
Fax Number:

Specialty:
Name:
Address:
Phone Number:
Fax Number:

Specialty:
Name:
Address:
Phone Number:
Fax Number:

Specialty:
Name:
Address:
Phone Number:
Fax Number:

{PHYSICIAN CONTACT LIST}

Specialty:
Name:
Address:
Phone Number:
Fax Number:

Specialty:
Name:
Address:
Phone Number:
Fax Number:

Specialty:
Name:
Address:
Phone Number:
Fax Number:

Specialty:
Name:
Address:
Phone Number:
Fax Number:

{PHYSICIAN CONTACT LIST}

Specialty:
Name:
Address:
Phone Number:
Fax Number:

Specialty:
Name:
Address:
Phone Number:
Fax Number:

Specialty:
Name:
Address:
Phone Number:
Fax Number:

Specialty:
Name:
Address:
Phone Number:
Fax Number:

{PHYSICIAN CONTACT LIST}

Specialty:
Name:
Address:
Phone Number:
Fax Number:

Specialty:
Name:
Address:
Phone Number:
Fax Number:

Specialty:
Name:
Address:
Phone Number:
Fax Number:

Specialty:
Name:
Address:
Phone Number:
Fax Number:

{PHYSICIAN CONTACT LIST}

Specialty:
Name:
Address:
Phone Number:
Fax Number:

Specialty:
Name:
Address:
Phone Number:
Fax Number:

Specialty:
Name:
Address:
Phone Number:
Fax Number:

Specialty:
Name:
Address:
Phone Number:
Fax Number:

{PHYSICIAN CONTACT LIST}

Specialty:
Name:
Address:
Phone Number:
Fax Number:

Specialty:
Name:
Address:
Phone Number:
Fax Number:

Specialty:
Name:
Address:
Phone Number:
Fax Number:

Specialty:
Name:
Address:
Phone Number:
Fax Number:

{PHYSICIAN CONTACT LIST}

Specialty:
Name:
Address:
Phone Number:
Fax Number:

Specialty:
Name:
Address:
Phone Number:
Fax Number:

Specialty:
Name:
Address:
Phone Number:
Fax Number:

Specialty:
Name:
Address:
Phone Number:
Fax Number:

{PHYSICIAN CONTACT LIST}

Specialty:
Name:
Address:
Phone Number:
Fax Number:

Specialty:
Name:
Address:
Phone Number:
Fax Number:

Specialty:
Name:
Address:
Phone Number:
Fax Number:

Specialty:
Name:
Address:
Phone Number:
Fax Number:

{PHYSICIAN CONTACT LIST}

Specialty:
Name:
Address:
Phone Number:
Fax Number:

Specialty:
Name:
Address:
Phone Number:
Fax Number:

Specialty:
Name:
Address:
Phone Number:
Fax Number:

Specialty:
Name:
Address:
Phone Number:
Fax Number:

{FAMILY MEDICAL HISTORY LOG SHEET}

Date: _____ Name: _____ Date of Birth _____

Family Member Name	
Relationship	
Date of Birth/Age	
Allergies	
Cause of Death	
Hereditary Illness or Medical Conditions:	

Family Member Name	
Relationship	
Date of Birth/Age	
Allergies	
Cause of Death	
Hereditary Illness or Medical Conditions:	

{FAMILY MEDICAL HISTORY LOG SHEET}

Date: _____ Name: _____ Date of Birth _____

Family Member Name	
Relationship	
Date of Birth/Age	
Allergies	
Cause of Death	
Hereditary Illness or Medical Conditions:	

Family Member Name	
Relationship	
Date of Birth/Age	
Allergies	
Cause of Death	
Hereditary Illness or Medical Conditions:	

{FAMILY MEDICAL HISTORY LOG SHEET}

Date: _____ Name: _____ Date of Birth _____

Family Member Name	
Relationship	
Date of Birth/Age	
Allergies	
Cause of Death	
Hereditary Illness or Medical Conditions:	

Family Member Name	
Relationship	
Date of Birth/Age	
Allergies	
Cause of Death	
Hereditary Illness or Medical Conditions:	

{FAMILY MEDICAL HISTORY LOG SHEET}

Date: _____ Name: _____ Date of Birth_____

Family Member Name	
Relationship	
Date of Birth/Age	
Allergies	
Cause of Death	
Hereditary Illness or Medical Conditions:	

Family Member Name	
Relationship	
Date of Birth/Age	
Allergies	
Cause of Death	
Hereditary Illness or Medical Conditions:	

{FAMILY MEDICAL HISTORY LOG SHEET}

Date: _____ Name: _____ Date of Birth _____

Family Member Name	
Relationship	
Date of Birth/Age	
Allergies	
Cause of Death	
Hereditary Illness or Medical Conditions:	

Family Member Name	
Relationship	
Date of Birth/Age	
Allergies	
Cause of Death	
Hereditary Illness or Medical Conditions:	

{FAMILY MEDICAL HISTORY LOG SHEET}

Date: _____ Name: _____ Date of Birth _____

Family Member Name	
Relationship	
Date of Birth/Age	
Allergies	
Cause of Death	
Hereditary Illness or Medical Conditions:	

Family Member Name	
Relationship	
Date of Birth/Age	
Allergies	
Cause of Death	
Hereditary Illness or Medical Conditions:	

{MEDICAL CONDITIONS CURRENTLY BEING TREATED}

Date: _____   Name: _____   D.O.B: _____

Current Medical Conditions Being Treated

Diagnosis	Prescriptions for Condition/Diagnosis

{MEDICAL CONDITIONS CURRENTLY BEING TREATED}

Date: _____ Name: _____ D.O.B: _____

Current Medical Conditions Being Treated

Diagnosis	Prescriptions for Condition/Diagnosis

{MEDICAL CONDITIONS CURRENTLY BEING TREATED}

Date: _____   Name: _____   D.O.B: _____

Current Medical Conditions Being Treated

Diagnosis	Prescriptions for Condition/Diagnosis

{MEDICAL CONDITIONS CURRENTLY BEING TREATED}

Date: _____   Name: _____   D.O.B: _____

Current Medical Conditions Being Treated

Diagnosis	Prescriptions for Condition/Diagnosis

{MEDICAL CONDITIONS CURRENTLY BEING TREATED}

Date: _____ Name: _____ D.O.B: _____

Current Medical Conditions Being Treated

Diagnosis	Prescriptions for Condition/Diagnosis

{MEDICAL CONDITIONS CURRENTLY BEING TREATED}

Date: _____ Name: _____ D.O.B: _____

Current Medical Conditions Being Treated

Diagnosis	Prescriptions for Condition/Diagnosis

{MEDICATION LOG SHEET}

Medication	
Frequency	
Dosage	
Purpose	

Medication	
Frequency	
Dosage	
Purpose	

Medication	
Frequency	
Dosage	
Purpose	

Medication	
Frequency	
Dosage	
Purpose	

Medication	
Frequency	
Dosage	
Purpose	

{MEDICATION LOG SHEET}

Medication	
Frequency	
Dosage	
Purpose	

Medication	
Frequency	
Dosage	
Purpose	

Medication	
Frequency	
Dosage	
Purpose	

Medication	
Frequency	
Dosage	
Purpose	

Medication	
Frequency	
Dosage	
Purpose	

{MEDICATION LOG SHEET}

Medication	
Frequency	
Dosage	
Purpose	

Medication	
Frequency	
Dosage	
Purpose	

Medication	
Frequency	
Dosage	
Purpose	

Medication	
Frequency	
Dosage	
Purpose	

Medication	
Frequency	
Dosage	
Purpose	

{MEDICATION LOG SHEET}

Medication	
Frequency	
Dosage	
Purpose	

Medication	
Frequency	
Dosage	
Purpose	

Medication	
Frequency	
Dosage	
Purpose	

Medication	
Frequency	
Dosage	
Purpose	

Medication	
Frequency	
Dosage	
Purpose	

{MEDICATION LOG SHEET}

Medication	
Frequency	
Dosage	
Purpose	

Medication	
Frequency	
Dosage	
Purpose	

Medication	
Frequency	
Dosage	
Purpose	

Medication	
Frequency	
Dosage	
Purpose	

Medication	
Frequency	
Dosage	
Purpose	

{MEDICATION LOG SHEET}

Medication	
Frequency	
Dosage	
Purpose	

Medication	
Frequency	
Dosage	
Purpose	

Medication	
Frequency	
Dosage	
Purpose	

Medication	
Frequency	
Dosage	
Purpose	

Medication	
Frequency	
Dosage	
Purpose	

{MEDICATION LOG SHEET}

Medication	
Frequency	
Dosage	
Purpose	

Medication	
Frequency	
Dosage	
Purpose	

Medication	
Frequency	
Dosage	
Purpose	

Medication	
Frequency	
Dosage	
Purpose	

Medication	
Frequency	
Dosage	
Purpose	

{MEDICATION LOG SHEET}

Medication	
Frequency	
Dosage	
Purpose	

Medication	
Frequency	
Dosage	
Purpose	

Medication	
Frequency	
Dosage	
Purpose	

Medication	
Frequency	
Dosage	
Purpose	

Medication	
Frequency	
Dosage	
Purpose	

{MEDICATION LOG SHEET}

Medication	
Frequency	
Dosage	
Purpose	

Medication	
Frequency	
Dosage	
Purpose	

Medication	
Frequency	
Dosage	
Purpose	

Medication	
Frequency	
Dosage	
Purpose	

Medication	
Frequency	
Dosage	
Purpose	

{MEDICATION LOG SHEET}

Medication	
Frequency	
Dosage	
Purpose	

Medication	
Frequency	
Dosage	
Purpose	

Medication	
Frequency	
Dosage	
Purpose	

Medication	
Frequency	
Dosage	
Purpose	

Medication	
Frequency	
Dosage	
Purpose	

{MEDICATION LOG SHEET}

Medication	
Frequency	
Dosage	
Purpose	

Medication	
Frequency	
Dosage	
Purpose	

Medication	
Frequency	
Dosage	
Purpose	

Medication	
Frequency	
Dosage	
Purpose	

Medication	
Frequency	
Dosage	
Purpose	

{ALLERGY LOG SHEET}

{Log Sheet for All Medications, Foods, etc. that you are allergic to}

ALLERGY	REACTION

{ALLERGY LOG SHEET}

{Log Sheet for All Medications, Foods, etc. that you are allergic to}

ALLERGY	REACTION

{ALLERGY LOG SHEET}

{Log Sheet for All Medications, Foods, etc. that you are allergic to}

ALLERGY	REACTION

{DOCTOR APPOINTMENT & FOLLOW-UP APPOINTMENT LOG SHEET}

{APPOINTMENT}

DATE	
DOCTOR	
Clinic/Hospital	
Reason For Follow-Up	
Special Instructions	

{FOLLOW-UP APPOINTMENT}

DATE	
DOCTOR	
Clinic/Hospital	
Reason For Follow-Up	
Special Instructions	

COMMENTS

{DOCTOR APPOINTMENT & FOLLOW-UP APPOINTMENT LOG SHEET}

{APPOINTMENT}

DATE	
DOCTOR	
Clinic/Hospital	
Reason For Follow-Up	
Special Instructions	

{FOLLOW-UP APPOINTMENT}

DATE	
DOCTOR	
Clinic/Hospital	
Reason For Follow-Up	
Special Instructions	

COMMENTS

{DOCTOR APPOINTMENT & FOLLOW-UP APPOINTMENT LOG SHEET}

{APPOINTMENT}

DATE	
DOCTOR	
Clinic/Hospital	
Reason For Follow-Up	
Special Instructions	

{FOLLOW-UP APPOINTMENT}

DATE	
DOCTOR	
Clinic/Hospital	
Reason For Follow-Up	
Special Instructions	

COMMENTS

{DOCTOR APPOINTMENT & FOLLOW-UP APPOINTMENT LOG SHEET}

{APPOINTMENT}

DATE	
DOCTOR	
Clinic/Hospital	
Reason For Follow-Up	
Special Instructions	

{FOLLOW-UP APPOINTMENT}

DATE	
DOCTOR	
Clinic/Hospital	
Reason For Follow-Up	
Special Instructions	

COMMENTS

{DOCTOR APPOINTMENT & FOLLOW-UP APPOINTMENT LOG SHEET}

{APPOINTMENT}

DATE	
DOCTOR	
Clinic/Hospital	
Reason For Follow-Up	
Special Instructions	

{FOLLOW-UP APPOINTMENT}

DATE	
DOCTOR	
Clinic/Hospital	
Reason For Follow-Up	
Special Instructions	

COMMENTS

{DOCTOR APPOINTMENT & FOLLOW-UP APPOINTMENT LOG SHEET}

{APPOINTMENT}

DATE	
DOCTOR	
Clinic/Hospital	
Reason For Follow-Up	
Special Instructions	

{FOLLOW-UP APPOINTMENT}

DATE	
DOCTOR	
Clinic/Hospital	
Reason For Follow-Up	
Special Instructions	

COMMENTS

{DOCTOR APPOINTMENT & FOLLOW-UP APPOINTMENT LOG SHEET}

{APPOINTMENT}

DATE	
DOCTOR	
Clinic/Hospital	
Reason For Follow-Up	
Special Instructions	

{FOLLOW-UP APPOINTMENT}

DATE	
DOCTOR	
Clinic/Hospital	
Reason For Follow-Up	
Special Instructions	

COMMENTS

{DOCTOR APPOINTMENT & FOLLOW-UP APPOINTMENT LOG SHEET}

{APPOINTMENT}

DATE	
DOCTOR	
Clinic/Hospital	
Reason For Follow-Up	
Special Instructions	

{FOLLOW-UP APPOINTMENT}

DATE	
DOCTOR	
Clinic/Hospital	
Reason For Follow-Up	
Special Instructions	

COMMENTS

{DOCTOR APPOINTMENT & FOLLOW-UP APPOINTMENT LOG SHEET}

{APPOINTMENT}

DATE	
DOCTOR	
Clinic/Hospital	
Reason For Follow-Up	
Special Instructions	

{FOLLOW-UP APPOINTMENT}

DATE	
DOCTOR	
Clinic/Hospital	
Reason For Follow-Up	
Special Instructions	

COMMENTS

{DOCTOR APPOINTMENT & FOLLOW-UP APPOINTMENT LOG SHEET}

{APPOINTMENT}

DATE	
DOCTOR	
Clinic/Hospital	
Reason For Follow-Up	
Special Instructions	

{FOLLOW-UP APPOINTMENT}

DATE	
DOCTOR	
Clinic/Hospital	
Reason For Follow-Up	
Special Instructions	

COMMENTS

{DOCTOR APPOINTMENT & FOLLOW-UP APPOINTMENT LOG SHEET}

{APPOINTMENT}

DATE	
DOCTOR	
Clinic/Hospital	
Reason For Follow-Up	
Special Instructions	

{FOLLOW-UP APPOINTMENT}

DATE	
DOCTOR	
Clinic/Hospital	
Reason For Follow-Up	
Special Instructions	

COMMENTS

{DOCTOR APPOINTMENT & FOLLOW-UP APPOINTMENT LOG SHEET}

{APPOINTMENT}

DATE	
DOCTOR	
Clinic/Hospital	
Reason For Follow-Up	
Special Instructions	

{FOLLOW-UP APPOINTMENT}

DATE	
DOCTOR	
Clinic/Hospital	
Reason For Follow-Up	
Special Instructions	

COMMENTS

{DOCTOR APPOINTMENT & FOLLOW-UP APPOINTMENT LOG SHEET}

{APPOINTMENT}

DATE	
DOCTOR	
Clinic/Hospital	
Reason For Follow-Up	
Special Instructions	

{FOLLOW-UP APPOINTMENT}

DATE	
DOCTOR	
Clinic/Hospital	
Reason For Follow-Up	
Special Instructions	

COMMENTS

{DOCTOR APPOINTMENT & FOLLOW-UP APPOINTMENT LOG SHEET}

{APPOINTMENT}

DATE	
DOCTOR	
Clinic/Hospital	
Reason For Follow-Up	
Special Instructions	

{FOLLOW-UP APPOINTMENT}

DATE	
DOCTOR	
Clinic/Hospital	
Reason For Follow-Up	
Special Instructions	

COMMENTS

{DOCTOR APPOINTMENT & FOLLOW-UP APPOINTMENT LOG SHEET}

{APPOINTMENT}

DATE	
DOCTOR	
Clinic/Hospital	
Reason For Follow-Up	
Special Instructions	

{FOLLOW-UP APPOINTMENT}

DATE	
DOCTOR	
Clinic/Hospital	
Reason For Follow-Up	
Special Instructions	

COMMENTS

{DOCTOR APPOINTMENT & FOLLOW-UP APPOINTMENT LOG SHEET}

{APPOINTMENT}

DATE	
DOCTOR	
Clinic/Hospital	
Reason For Follow-Up	
Special Instructions	

{FOLLOW-UP APPOINTMENT}

DATE	
DOCTOR	
Clinic/Hospital	
Reason For Follow-Up	
Special Instructions	

COMMENTS

{MEDICAL TEST LOG SHEET}

{What tests are you scheduled for? Log all your Outpatient Tests here}

DATE	TEST/SCAN/BIOPSY/MRI etc.	LOCATION OF TESTING

{MEDICAL TEST LOG SHEET}

{What tests are you scheduled for? Log all your Outpatient Tests here}

DATE	TEST/SCAN/BIOPSY/MRI etc.	LOCATION OF TESTING

{MEDICAL TEST LOG SHEET}

{What tests are you scheduled for? Log all your Outpatient Tests here}

DATE	TEST/SCAN/BIOPSY/MRI etc.	LOCATION OF TESTING

{MEDICAL TEST LOG SHEET}

{What tests are you scheduled for? Log all your Outpatient Tests here}

DATE	TEST/SCAN/BIOPSY/MRI etc.	LOCATION OF TESTING

{MEDICAL TEST LOG SHEET}

{What tests are you scheduled for? Log all your Outpatient Tests here}

DATE	TEST/SCAN/BIOPSY/MRI etc.	LOCATION OF TESTING

{MEDICAL TEST LOG SHEET}

{What tests are you scheduled for? Log all your Outpatient Tests here}

DATE	TEST/SCAN/BIOPSY/MRI etc.	LOCATION OF TESTING

{MEDICAL TEST LOG SHEET}

{What tests are you scheduled for? Log all your Outpatient Tests here}

DATE	TEST/SCAN/BIOPSY/MRI etc.	LOCATION OF TESTING

{MEDICAL TEST LOG SHEET}

{What tests are you scheduled for? Log all your Outpatient Tests here}

DATE	TEST/SCAN/BIOPSY/MRI etc.	LOCATION OF TESTING

{MEDICAL TEST LOG SHEET}

{What tests are you scheduled for? Log all your Outpatient Tests here}

DATE	TEST/SCAN/BIOPSY/MRI etc.	LOCATION OF TESTING

{MEDICAL TEST LOG SHEET}

{What tests are you scheduled for? Log all your Outpatient Tests here}

DATE	TEST/SCAN/BIOPSY/MRI etc.	LOCATION OF TESTING

{MEDICAL TEST LOG SHEET}

{What tests are you scheduled for? Log all your Outpatient Tests here}

DATE	TEST/SCAN/BIOPSY/MRI etc.	LOCATION OF TESTING

{ADDITIONAL NOTES/ COMMENTS/ CONCERNS}

{ADDITIONAL NOTES/ COMMENTS/ CONCERNS}

{ADDITIONAL NOTES/ COMMENTS/ CONCERNS}

{ADDITIONAL NOTES/ COMMENTS/ CONCERNS}

{ADDITIONAL NOTES/ COMMENTS/ CONCERNS}

{ADDITIONAL NOTES/ COMMENTS/ CONCERNS}

{ADDITIONAL NOTES/ COMMENTS/ CONCERNS}

{ADDITIONAL NOTES/ COMMENTS/ CONCERNS}

{ADDITIONAL NOTES/ COMMENTS/ CONCERNS}

{ADDITIONAL NOTES/ COMMENTS/ CONCERNS}

{ADDITIONAL NOTES/ COMMENTS/ CONCERNS}

Printed in the USA
CPSIA information can be obtained
at www.ICGtesting.com
LVHW070303041024
792850LV00032B/740